PENGUIN BOOKS

5 MINUTES A DAY

Michelle Bridges became a household name when she first appeared as a trainer on Channel Ten's hit reality weight-loss show *The Biggest Loser*. She is now Australia's most recognised personal trainer, having worked in the fitness and weight-loss industry for over two decades. Michelle is also highly sought after as a motivational speaker.

Her first three books, *Crunch Time*, *Crunch Time Cookbook* and *Losing the Last 5 Kilos*, were bestsellers, with *Losing the Last 5 Kilos* debuting at number 1 nationally.

5 MINUTES A DAY

simple tips for weight-loss and wellbeing

michelle bridges

PENGUIN BOOKS

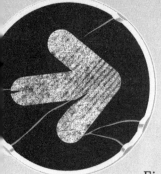

INTRODUCTION

SOMETIMES ALL IT TAKES IS 5 MINUTES A DAY.

Five minutes to think about where you are in relation to your goals. Five minutes to plan your eating. Five minutes to plan your exercise. Five minutes of exercise, walking to the bus or train stop. Five minutes to make a great salad for lunch. Five minutes of working out how you're going to get where you want to go – and what you're going to do about it **TODAY!**

Every minute counts, especially when you remember that all those minutes add up to a lifetime. And I want you to get the best out of your life.

HERE'S HOW YOU CAN DO IT.

This book is designed to be opened at any page – **FLICK THROUGH AND STOP!** There will be a message for your day and it might be exactly what you need to hear!

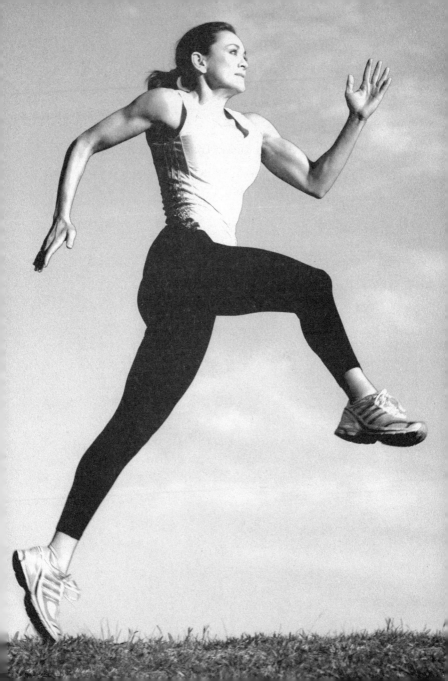

To all my fitness industry colleagues and clients,
who have taught me valuable lessons along the way

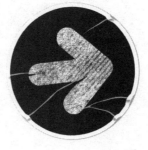

Thoughts.
Words.
Then

ACTION.

SELF-AWARENESS

is the first step to change.

MOTIVATION IS LIKE A BAD BOYFRIEND...

never there when you need him.

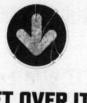

GET OVER IT!

Turn up and be consistent!

Do you hear yourself saying or thinking things like,

'IT'S NOT MY FAULT'

'IF I HAD HER LIFE IT WOULD BE EASIER'

'WHY IS THIS HAPPENING TO ME?'

'IT'S NOT FAIR!'

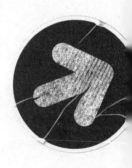

Then **YOU'RE** buying into

BEING A VICTIM.

We've all done it at one time or another, but those of you who live by it consistently relinquish **ALL OF YOUR POWER!**

If you're a victim, then of course you must have 'villains' in your life – the villains are the people or circumstances to whom you are giving all your power! **TAKE BACK YOUR POWER** by being someone who chooses to act and think differently. Take a mature approach to what you want.

Have you ever given a child a lolly to pacify them? To cheer them up? To stop them from crying? Make them feel better?

COULD THIS BE THE START OF EMOTIONAL EATING?

I say **YES!** Do this enough times and you'll lay down some very strong habits – habits that can **FOLLOW YOUR KIDS** into adult life.

When you change your diet, exercise and environment, there's an immediate change to your **GENE EXPRESSION** (the way your genetic code is interpreted in your body). Never think that the changes you've made to your lifestyle haven't made a difference –

THEY HAVE!

And the difference took place at a cellular level

THE MOMENT YOU MADE THE CHANGE.

So don't be disheartened – every single healthy choice you make improves your overall health **STRAIGHT AWAY!**

J.F.D.I.

('just f***ing do it')

This is the card I pull out when I'm whinging
and moaning about having to train
(yes, it happens to the best of us).
Sometimes you need to cut the crap,
shut the hell up and **J.F.D.I!**

Sometimes when I don't feel like training, my thoughts go something like this:

I CAN DO IT THIS AFTERNOON

I HAVE TOO MUCH ON

THERE'S NOT REALLY ENOUGH TIME TO MAKE IT WORTHWHILE

. . . blah, blah, blah.

Yep, we've all been there before, right? And **IT'S 100 PER CENT ALL IN YOUR HEAD.** Stop procrastinating. Stop thinking about it. Just get out there and do it.

It's crazy really – **WE ALL KNOW WHAT WE SHOULD BE EATING.**

There are no secrets out there. How many times have you heard someone say, 'I shouldn't be eating this, but . . . ' as they stuff another piece of banana bread into their mouth? **DOES THIS SOUND FAMILIAR?**

We all pretty much know **WHAT WE SHOULD – AND SHOULDN'T –** eat to maintain a healthy weight.

SHOW YOUR KIDS HOW TO EAT WELL,

keep junk food as an occasional treat, and you'll have given them

A HEADSTART ON LIFE.

Go get your wheelie bin from outside.
Bring it into the kitchen.

Open the pantry, fridge and freezer.

NOW, START CHUCKING!

THROW OUT EVERY

BIT OF CRAP FOOD

THAT'S HOLDING YOU BACK.

Maybe you think throwing out all the crap food in your fridge, freezer and pantry is a waste. Here's what I think is a waste – having all this **BAGGAGE** weighing you

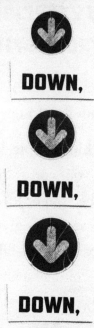

DOWN,

DOWN,

DOWN,

for years and years and years. Letting it hold you back from participating in life at every level. Letting it hold you back from being **YOU!**
NOW THAT'S A WASTE!

STRENGTHEN YOUR WILLPOWER MUSCLE.
Improving your willpower is a lot like improving your fitness –

THE MORE YOU EXERCISE IT
THE STRONGER IT BECOMES.

If your willpower needs a work-out, start exercising it in your day-to-day life.

Begin with something simple, like having only one sugar in your coffee instead of two, or getting out of bed ten or fifteen minutes earlier. Then you can tackle giving up things that are a bit more addictive, like cigarettes. Importantly, give yourself a pat on the back every time you say

'NO'.

I'm a major fan of habits and rituals.
(Of course, I'm talking about the ones that are good for us.) They keep us consistent, and we all know **CONSISTENCY IS KING,** right? Think about it. When was the last time you had to psych yourself up to brush your teeth?

Do something long enough and consistently enough and **IT WILL BECOME SECOND NATURE.**

GET IT?

Paralysis by analysis! Is this you?

ARE YOU OVER-THINKING IT?

'Should I train in the morning? The evening?',
'Should I eat before or after training?',
'Do I have the right runners?', 'Is this bra too
baggy?', 'Should I stretch first?', 'Could I be
dehydrated?', 'Maybe it's too cold; I might
get a headache', 'My astrologer said I'll train
better when my lunar sun is in my Libra
rising moon . . .'

SHUT UP AND GET ON WITH IT!

Cravings are like emotions: joy, anger, happiness, sorrow, boredom, fear, excitement. We can experience tons of different feelings in a single day – and cravings come and go just as frequently.

If we understand that

A CRAVING WILL PASS,

like a wave in the ocean, can we not simply ride it out?

ARE YOU A SELF-SABOTEUR?

Do you derail yourself when you're on track and achieving results? You're not alone. Understand, though, that **IT IS PRECONCEIVED.** A Cherry Ripe (or three) doesn't just fall into your mouth! No, you've actually thought it through – where you'll buy the Cherry Ripes, how many you'll get and when you'll eat them – all the while justifying that you deserve it, have earned it and worked for it.

The time between when you think of the (bad) idea and when you start to act is crucial! That's when your inner adult needs to show up. Are you a woman or man of your word? What exactly will this old habit achieve?

THINK IT THROUGH!

Picture the end results – goodness knows, you've seen them many times before.

You know how this story ends. So stop lying to yourself and saying, 'I don't know how it happens or why I do it.' I challenge you and say, 'Yes you do! On both fronts!' I say this with love –

IT'S TIME TO GROW UP.

We're all totally preoccupied with how we look, yet it's easy to forget how our bodies are **ACTUALLY FUNCTIONING.** We tend to forget that we are the manifestation of what we do to our bodies –

OUR PHYSICAL SELVES ARE MERELY A REFLECTION OF OUR LIFESTYLES.

So whilst we might think that we're stuck with a certain physical body, we're not.

WE CAN CHANGE IT

by giving it different messages. Now, nothing happens **OVERNIGHT.** Your body is a long time in the making, and it's not quick to change. But change it will, because your body responds perfectly to what you tell it to do.

Check in. And be **BRUTALLY HONEST.**

When was the last time you claimed you were going to clean up your act, drop a few kilos and get fitter, only to blow off your second training session and help yourself to a second slice of chocolate cake at the office party three days in? The truth is, while you think it'd be nice to lose weight, it's just not that important to you.

IT'S NOT HIGH ENOUGH OF A PRIORITY.

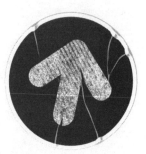

Do you have a

FEAR OF SUCCESS?

One of my female clients told me she was worried that if she lost weight she'd become more attractive to the opposite sex, which for her would be very **STRESSFUL.** Another woman told me that she felt she'd have to compete with other women if she lost weight – again, a stressful situation.

Do you have a

FEAR OF FAILURE?

A female client of mine shared with me that she couldn't stand going through it 'again' – the whole yoyo diet thing had destroyed her confidence.

And yet, with further investigation, she didn't have a fear of failure. **NO.** That was camouflage. Her real fear was the

FEAR OF COMMITMENT
AND RESPONSIBILITY.

She was afraid of having to eat healthy food most of the time, do regular exercise and be accountable for it! Wow – big breakthrough! If you can relate, it's time to do an analysis of the costs and payoffs.

COSTS AND PAYOFFS ANALYSIS.

Draw up a table with two columns, and write 'COSTS' at the top of one and 'PAYOFFS' at the top of the other. Now ask yourself, 'What do I get out of being overweight? What are the kickbacks, the pay-offs, the perks?' Dig deep here. Don't hold anything back – in fact, the things you want to hold back should go at the top of the list!

Do the same for the costs: what is being overweight costing you? Then, **WEIGH UP THE TWO COLUMNS . . .**

There's a difference between having to do something and choosing to do it. You feel burdened when you have to do it, but

YOU FEEL FREE

WHEN YOU CHOOSE TO.

You're at a crossroad.

YOU EITHER CHOOSE IT

OR YOU DON'T.

Do yourself and everyone around you a favour – don't say you will if you know you won't! The key is to be truly okay with whatever **CHOICE** you make.

PUT ON YOUR OWN OXYGEN MASK
BEFORE HELPING
THOSE AROUND YOU.

I remind all the mums I work with of these airline safety instructions. There's a clear message here: unless you take care of yourself first,

YOU ARE NO USE TO ANYONE.

What's the point of ruining your make-up crying if you don't learn something from the experience?

STOP REPEATING YOUR MISTAKES.

Unless you're prepared to make a change in

THE PRESENT,

YOUR FUTURE

CAN ONLY REFLECT YOUR PAST.

TALKING is good,
but it should be setting
the stage for **ACTION,**

NOT REPLACING IT!

Losing weight is a

SCIENCE.

Keeping it off is

PSYCHOLOGY.

The two are completely different.

MAKE A LIST OF ALL THE THINGS YOU NEED TO DO.

Absolutely everything – sorting out drawers, downloading photos, calling back a friend. It's long, right?

These are now the things you can do instead of going to the fridge. Better yet, stick the list on the fridge – along with a current photo of you in a

BIKINI!

BE CONSISTENT.

This is one of my golden tips! It covers everything from food choices, to exercise, to the way you think.

BE YOUR WORD.

Have integrity around the choices you've made for yourself, and watch your inner warrior grow.

UNDERSTAND YOURSELF.

If you know that an all-you-can-eat buffet turns you into Homer Simpson, **DON'T GO TO ONE!** If you know you have to train in the mornings, because you never do it in the evening even when you tell yourself you will, get to bed earlier and **GET IT DONE!** If you know that you make dumb food choices when you drink, then don't drink – be the designated driver instead. When you know yourself, you can **SAVE YOURSELF A LOT OF TORMENT.**

Have you ever turned to food to **CHEER** yourself up, to **RELEASE STRESS** or as a **REWARD?**

UM, HELLO?

Is anyone out there joining the dots?

Put things on lay-by – we never do this anymore, do we? It's all about having stuff instantly. Next time you hear yourself very maturely saying, 'But I have to have that chocolate bar **NOW!**' I want you to go into

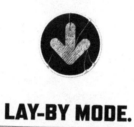

LAY-BY MODE.

TAKE A 24-HOUR COOLING-OFF PERIOD.

If after 24 hours you still want the damn bar, have it! But add it into your daily calorie quota. This way, you're not giving into your own childish demands and handing your power over to the chocolate. Instead, you are **TAKING CONTROL** by choosing when you'll eat it –

POWER BACK!

BREAK OLD HABITS

WITH NEW HABITS.

Give them some time: they'll soon settle in.

Don't let your ego get in the way of being the best version of yourself, at any age.

WHO CARES IF YOU WON'T BE

THE FASTEST?

THE BEST?

THE WINNER?

Really. Give up the ego and be a winner by participating.

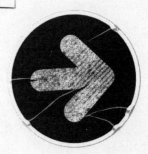

Stop living off past achievements! If you're still **LANGUISHING IN YOUR GLORY DAYS,** saying, 'I was so fit when I was eighteen . . .' you're dreaming. That was then, this is now –

SO LET'S GET MOVING!

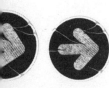

YOU GOTTA HAVE A PLAN, MAN!

It's knowing **HOW** you're going to get there that makes it happen. Weigh yourself, measure yourself, take a photo of yourself, set a goal or two and then **EXECUTE IT WITH MILITARY PRECISION.** Mark it up on your calendar, set up shopping lists, meal plans and an exercise routine. Oh, and be consistent. I'm not talking three days here – this is a **LIFETIME COMMITMENT!**

THE POWER OF
LANGUAGE IS EXTRAORDINARY.

Remove everything from your self-talk that's
NEGATIVE about you and your ability –
then start telling yourself the reverse.
What you think and say will be.

It's your

MIND

that has got your

BODY

where it is today.

Self-control equals

SELF-RESPECT.

Why is it that we eat like **TEENAGERS** whose parents have gone away for the weekend?

USE A SHOPPING LIST when you go shopping – it'll keep you on track and focused. It's also a good idea **NOT** to be starving when you go, and avoid all aisles which contain crap food. Don't tempt fate.

Oh, and be sure not to take your **INNER TEENAGER** with you. Lock 'em in their bedroom –

FOR LIFE!

There is no way on this planet you can accelerate yourself to

 LEAN AND MEAN

unless you put some time into **YOUR KITCHEN.** Get some recipes under your belt and throw out the takeaway menus.

Let me tell you, **THERE ARE ENTIRE SUPERMARKET AISLES** that you must never go down again if you're to reach your **GOAL!**

Losing weight will always come down to

WHAT YOU PUT IN YOUR MOUTH.

END OF STORY!

If I had two clients,

one of whom refused to eat well but trained like a demon every day,

and another who did no exercise but cleaned up her **DIET** so that she had a weekly calorie deficit,

THE NON-EXERCISER
WOULD LOSE THE MOST WEIGHT.

You know what? For the most part,
PEOPLE JUST EAT TOO MUCH.

PERIOD.

Are you someone who **REGULARLY USES FOOD TO COMFORT YOURSELF?**
As a reward? To make yourself happy?
To relieve boredom? To celebrate? As revenge?
To manipulate? So you have something to
look forward to?

The key word in that question is

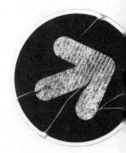

'REGULARLY'.

Some of these are very normal behaviours; however, when they're taken to the **EXTREME** and done every day, in my mind, there's a deeper power at work. I truly believe that to find the answers **YOU NEED TO DO SOME SOLID INTROSPECTION.**

This is where a professional therapist could be worth their weight in gold.

NEVER GO BACK FOR SECONDS.

It's a habit which will serve you poorly,
as you're training yourself and your stomach
to want more.

NEVER EAT THE LEFTOVERS

from the children's dinner.

Your **KITCHEN** is ground control in the

WAR ON WEIGHT LOSS.

Personally, as someone who's at their goal weight, I tend to stick to a clean, healthy nutrition plan during the week and **RELAX THE REINS ON THE WEEKEND.** I still train on the weekend, though. And I said **'RELAX'** the reins, not sever them with a carving knife and let the horse bolt!

IT'S NORMAL AND NECESSARY to allow yourself to eat your favourite foods. But what makes them so special AND enjoyable is that you don't have them all the time. You look forward to them and **SAVOUR THEM** when you eat them,

GUILT-FREE!

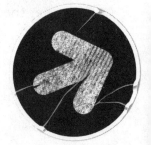

Compare this with the alternative – eating those foods **EVERY DAY,** always feeling guilty afterwards, always feeling tired, putting on weight and running the health risks that come with it . . . I'd honestly have to

QUESTION YOUR SANITY

if you keep doing that!

If your primary goal is to **LOSE WEIGHT,**
then your primary concern should be

THE NUMBER OF CALORIES YOU EAT.

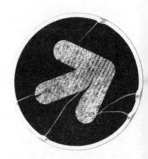

HOW MANY CALORIES SHOULD YOU EAT?

I tend to set my weight-loss candidates a quota – 1200 calories a day for my girls and 1800 calories a day for my guys. They get a meal on the weekend when they can splurge (usually Saturday dinner), but they must train that day and eat lightly at the other meals.

Set up your **'EATING WEEK'** much the same as your 'exercise week'. For example, at my house:

- Monday night is stir-fry night

- Tuesday night is fish night

- Wednesday night is soup night

- Thursday night is steak night

- Friday night is homemade pizza night

- Saturday night we eat out (and I'm relaxed about my choices)

- Sunday night is poached chicken night – and I make extra portions for lunches during the week.

Having a plan like this

TAKES THE THINKING OUT OF IT

and helps you avoid the potential pitfalls.

Foods that are good for you
NUTRITIONALLY
just happen to also be
LOW in calories.

GO FIGURE!

MY SNOWBALL THEORY.

You know the cartoon where a snowball starts rolling down a mountain and gets faster and faster and bigger and bigger? That's what your **METABOLISM** is like once you get it up and running with regular exercise and good nutrition.

If you have one **TREAT MEAL** each week, it's a bit like a single tree standing up in the snow – when the snowball strikes, it takes the tree out no problem and just keeps rolling. The snowball does have a problem, however, if that **SINGLE TREE BECOMES A FOREST.**

ARE YOU HEARIN' ME?

Get to know the **CALORIES** in the food that you **REGULARLY EAT.** We tend to be creatures of habit, so if you understand how many calories are in the foods you eat often, it'll be easy to know if you're

or

 OVER

your quota.

A kilogram of body weight represents approximately 7000 calories. If you can

WIPE 7000 CALORIES

OUT OF YOUR WEEKLY DIET

you will start to see results.

ADD A BIT OF EXERCISE to that and you'll be very pleased with the outcome!

SNACKS are a great way to support weight management and weight loss, **BUT LET'S GET REAL.** A snack is a small portion of food, about 100–150 calories' worth,

NOT A MEAL LADEN

WITH SUGAR, SALT AND FAT!

Oh, and can you let go of all the emotion around snacks? You know the stuff . . .

DREAMING,

OBSESSING,

FIXATING,

attaching statements to them like, 'I can't live without it!' Yawn, bored now. Are the words

'GET A LIFE' too harsh?

Sometimes I'm only looking for a snack because I'm **BORED.** Ask yourself honestly: are you feeling **HUNGER PANGS,** or are you just trying to think of a reason to stop working and get away from your desk? If it's the latter, by all means go for a walk, but don't take any money with you!

If I had a dollar for every time someone said,

'I SHOULDN'T BE EATING THIS, BUT...'

I'd be a very rich woman.

Do you have **FRIENDS WHO UNWITTINGLY DISTRACT** you from your weight-loss goals? 'Go on, have another drink', 'Come on, let's get pizza.'

We have a responsibility to make ourselves happy, because no-one else can do it for us.

(WE HAVE TO PUT ON OUR OWN OXYGEN MASKS FIRST, REMEMBER?)

A 'responsibility' – our happiness or unhappiness is purely down to our 'ability' to 'respond' to what's going on around us. You can **CHOOSE TO RESPOND IN A WAY THAT EMPOWERS YOU** or in a way that disempowers you.

It's not them. **IT'S YOU!** Cool, huh?
We're the ones in control of our own feelings!

Next time you go to the gym, warm up, then do a 500-metre **SPRINT** on the rowing machine – then do your regular training session. Your work-out will be taken to another level.

ENJOY!

GET YOURSELF A HEART-RATE MONITOR.

I love using mine to play a few mind games with myself: 'Okay, Michelle, you cannot leave the gym until you have burnt 600 calories' or 'You must get your heart rate to 170 bpm, then you can let it come down to 130 bpm – but it's **GOTTA GO BACK UP AGAIN** after that!' Fun times, good memories!

If you enjoy classes at the gym (one of my favourite ways to train), then do all you can to

TURN UP EARLY

and jump on a cross trainer, treadmill or bike **BEFOREHAND.** You'll get more out of your class that way, as you'll have switched into 'training mode' –

YOU'LL BURN HEAPS MORE
CALORIES, TOO!

Nothing holds back the years like weight training! It really is the

FOUNTAIN OF YOUTH.

Have you measured your **WAIST** lately?
Grab a tape measure and do it

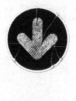

NOW.

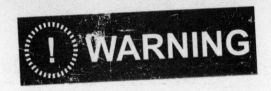

WOMEN

with a waist measurement of under 80 cm
are not considered to be at risk of

HEART DISEASE;

they have an increased risk if it's between
80 cm to 88 cm, and a substantially increased
risk if it's over 88 cm.

MEN

are not at risk with a waist circumference
of under 94 cm, but have an increased
risk between 94 cm and 102 cm, and a
substantially increased risk over 102 cm.

THE BODY MASS INDEX (BMI) WORKS!

There are some out there who believe it doesn't, simply because heavily muscled athletes like footballers rate as obese on the scale.

It's a flawed argument, though. Last time I checked,

ATHLETES AND BODY BUILDERS DIDN'T HAVE WEIGHT PROBLEMS.

It's the general public who do, and BMI works perfectly for them.

Always **HAVE A PLAN** before you train. Every time I turn up to the gym or for a workout session and have no plan, I have a wishy-washy session.

When I have a plan laid down, it takes the thinking out of it. When you're left to your own devices and have to think, I've discovered,

YOU USUALLY

JUST TALK YOURSELF OUT OF IT.

I get quizzed a lot about **OVERTRAINING,**
but I have to be blunt on this one –
Olympians, professional sportspeople,
yes, they can be at risk of overtraining.
**BUT THE AVERAGE OVERWEIGHT
AUSTRALIAN?** Ah . . . not too many
overtrainers out there. Anyone asking me
about overtraining is usually looking for an

EXCUSE NOT TO EXERCISE.

SUPER SATURDAYS

are my day to crank it up. I choose Saturday because I normally go out for dinner on Saturday night.

I knock out two hours of training, eat healthily but lightly throughout the day, and really enjoy my meal out – entree, main, wine and possibly even a shared dessert!

When you're **EATING OUT** for dinner with friends, make sure you have a healthy afternoon snack. Group dinners are notorious for having a big gap between ordering and dinner turning up – by then you've often

INHALED THE BREAD BASKET.

If you have to **EAT OUT FREQUENTLY** for work, ask questions about your meal, go for the

CLEAN, LIGHT OPTION

and tell them to take the bread basket away – or send it to the other end of the table.

Get a **TRAINING PARTNER.**

Find someone you can rely on, who wants to
make a difference to their training too, and

SHARE YOUR GOALS AND ASPIRATIONS

for training with each other.

That way, when you call them up to say you can't make a session, they can give you all the reasons **WHY** you're training, tell you to

SHUT THE HELL UP

and say they'll see you at 6 a.m. tomorrow!

LOVE IT!

One of the best and most rewarding ways to exercise is to get out there with your family and/or friends. Cycling, rollerblading, beach cricket, whatever –

IT'S FUN,

IT'S ACTIVE AND IT WORKS.

Bonus for those with kids – no adult ever lovingly recalls their childhood memories of sitting at home watching TV, but

MEMORIES OF PLAYING
WITH THEIR PARENTS?

PRICELESS.

Give a girl a set of boxing gloves and watch her **TRANSFORM!** Every female client I have ever introduced to boxing simply falls in **LOVE** with it. It's as though suddenly they have permission to **PUNCH,** and wow! How empowered are they after a great boxing session? As well as exhausted and

STRESS-FREE!

Why are you sitting up at night watching **MINDLESS TV** or trawling the internet with **NO REAL PURPOSE?**

GET TO BED!

SLEEP is a key ingredient in health, weight loss and **SANITY!** Try going to bed an hour earlier: you'll be amazed at how good you'll feel.

Take a look at the amazing machine
that is your body.

YES, IT IS AMAZING!

You might notice that your body is
jam-packed with moveable parts.
YOU ARE DESIGNED TO MOVE!
Your body loves it.

I'm talking about your body here,
not your head, so

DON'T GIVE ME ALL THAT BOLLOCKS
ABOUT NOT LIKING EXERCISE.

That's your head, not your body. Your body
LOVES TO MOVE! Switch your head off
and get out the door!

Grab your diary, sit down and **LOCK IN** your training times. This'll be the best five minutes you'll ever spend on your health.

You need about forty-five minutes, six days a week when you can commit to training. You won't 'find the time',

YOU MUST MAKE THE TIME.

BEST TIME OF DAY TO TRAIN?

First thing in the morning: it's when you're least likely to be pulled away from it, and you'll **GET THE MONKEY OFF YA BACK** nice and early.

INTERVAL TRAINING IS A GENIUS WAY TO EXERCISE. It can chew up stacks of calories and hit major muscle groups in a functional way (which is a really smart way to train) – and above all else, it keeps the mind busy!

There are no real rules with interval training. You can mix and match the body parts you're working, the modes of exercise and your time frames.

YOUR IMAGINATION IS THE ONLY THING HOLDING YOU BACK.

The key benefit to intervals is that

YOU GET MORE OUT OF YOURSELF.

If I asked you to go at 100 per cent intensity for sixty minutes, you'd tell me to go jump, right?

HOWEVER, if we set up a sequence of cardio or strength exercises and I ask you to go all out for only thirty seconds on each, then you'd probably give me more than you thought you had in you!

INTERVAL RUNNING ON THE TREADMILL is a favourite work-out of mine. I train my clients first at a walking pace, and build to a running pace once they've got some confidence. Thirty seconds on and thirty seconds off, with the treadmill being the timekeeper.

Ten rounds in ten minutes is a pretty good place to start: you can build up to longer durations as your **FITNESS INCREASES.**

CRANK THAT SNOOZY MOTOR UP
A GEAR first thing in the morning and you'll set yourself up for an elevated metabolism throughout the day.

Grab your skipping-rope and skip for one minute, then punch out twenty push-ups. Then go back to the skipping for a minute, followed by twenty crunches. Then skip for another minute before twenty more push-ups.

NONSTOP, GO FAST, FIVE MINUTES TOTAL.

If you enjoy one hour of TV viewing a night, then **YOU'VE JUST FOUND YOURSELF TWENTY MINUTES TO TRAIN** that you didn't know you had!

Every commercial, get up and bang out some exercise. Squats for the first ad, then push-ups, then hallway runs, then crunches – you can add a few more after that or start from the top and go again. If being time poor is your number-one excuse,

YOU JUST LOST IT.

Get a **CHECK-UP.** When was the last time you took yourself in to the GP for a full service? I bet your car has had more maintenance than you!

DON'T BE A BABY.

MAKE AN APPOINTMENT.

THE SEVEN-MINUTE RUN IS YOUR FRIEND!

Out of bed, joggers on and run away from your house as fast as you can for seven minutes. Then turn around and get home in eight minutes. You've got an extra minute up your sleeve on the way back, but if you went hard on the way out, trust me,

YOU'LL NEED IT!

Don't forget to wear your watch – and when it all gets a bit easy, pick a route with some hills.

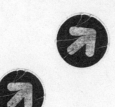

Warm up with the Seven-minute Run, then belt out this **KILLER CIRCUIT** before you go to work.

Six exercises, twenty repetitions each, **FIFTEEN MINUTES TOTAL.** It looks like this – skips, push-ups, frog jumps, tricep bench dips, lunges and finish with crunches.

Take a one-minute breather before starting again, and repeat until the fifteen minutes are up. Do this five times a week and

KICK THE SLUG

IN YOUR METABOLISM TO THE KERB!

FOR FLABBY ARMS.

PART ONE

FIVE MINUTES

You need to get your heart rate up to kiss
goodbye to those tuckshop arms, so you'll
want to move fast for this one.

Grab your kitchen chair and push it above your head twenty times. Then smash out twenty push-ups (on your toes preferably) followed by twenty tricep dips on your chair, before going back to the beginning and repeating the whole thing.

FIVE MINUTES, BALLS TO THE WALL, NO REST.

FOR FLABBY ARMS.

PART TWO
FIFTEEN MINUTES

Boxing rips everything. When was the last time you saw a fat boxer? So here's your circuit – one minute of head-high punches on the bag, then twenty shoulder presses with a light barbell. Back to the bag for one minute of body rips down low, then grab the barbell for twenty bicep curls.

Take a short break before repeating. If you can get through this circuit more than three times in fifteen minutes,

I WANT TO KNOW YOUR NAME!

FOR FLABBY ARMS.

PART THREE
THIRTY MINUTES

Time to hit the gym. Start with the rowing machine – warm up for two minutes before doing a 500-metre sprint. If you can do the sprint in less than two minutes,

YOU'RE SMOKIN'.

Next, five exercises for ten repetitions each. Start with assisted chin-ups (underhand grip), followed by chest presses, bicep curls, shoulder presses and tricep dips.

Take a minute's break, then repeat.

GO FAST,

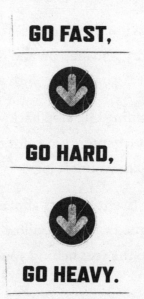

GO HARD,

GO HEAVY.

Grab a trainer if necessary to show you the exercises. And kiss those arms goodbye . . .

THE FIVE-MINUTE

NO BUTS BUTT WORK-OUT.

Perform twenty repetitions for each of these exercises:

- ➡ First, get a low bench or a seat that's about knee height, and step up and down with your right leg only, then with your left.

- ➡ Next, standing tall, step backward with your right leg into a lunge for twenty reps, then swap to your left leg.

- ➡ Lastly, do twenty squats above the bench, knees aligned with toes, allowing your butt to just tap the seat behind you.

THE FIFTEEN-MINUTE
NO BUTS BUTT WORK-OUT.

Step up on to a knee-height bench fifteen times with your right leg, then fifteen times with your left. Repeat this five times through without stopping. Do twenty squats, rest for thirty seconds, do another twenty squats. You need to squeeze in a five-minute run, either around the block or on a treadmill,

SO KEEP THE PACE FAST!

THE THIRTY-MINUTE
NO BUTS BUTT WORK-OUT.

Start with five minutes on the cross trainer and **GO HARD** for the last two.

Then alternate twenty barbell or freestanding squats with ten step-ups on each leg, three times through.

Next, find a low step, and step backwards into a lunge – twenty times each leg, three times through, with no rest in between sets if you can.

Then pump out twenty frog jumps up and down the room before getting back on the cross trainer for your final blast –

SPRINT TO THE FINISH LINE!

FIFTEEN-MINUTE

WOW-FACTOR WAISTLINE.

Ten minutes of running. Yep, that's right!
All the ab exercises under the sun ain't gonna
shift a wobbly stomach, so start huffing and
puffing!

After that, get stuck in to five minutes of
ab training. You can do any ab exercise you
like – straight crunches, twisting crunches –
but ya gotta do one hundred!

ONE HUNDRED!

MAY THE FORCE BE WITH YOU!

THIRTY-MINUTE
WOW-FACTOR WAISTLINE.

Run to your local park and set up a circuit of stairs, push-ups, fifteen-metre sprints, crunches, step-ups on a bench and twisting crunches.

Spend one minute at each station, and move from station to station with urgency. Go through the circuit as many times as you can, leaving enough time to jog home.

Remember, though, the **BIG** factor is what you put in your mouth, **SO DON'T BLOW ALL YOUR HARD WORK** by eating tons afterwards!

EPIGENETICS

– it's not the cards you're dealt,

IT'S HOW YOU PLAY THEM.

One of the things scientists are focusing their attention on at the moment is epigenetics, particularly now that we've unravelled the human genome. In the past, we've looked to our parents and grandparents for the determinants of the way we look, or our propensity for disease or obesity. What epigenetic research is telling us is that **OUR GENES ARE NOT WHOLLY RESPONSIBLE** for our physical characteristics.

We can't change our genetic sequence, because it's hardwired into us. But

WE CAN CHANGE OUR EPIGENETICS

– the way our genes express themselves (a.k.a. genetic expression).

And here's the amazing news. The way to change our epigenetics – our propensity to disease, obesity, even the way we look – is to change

OUR DIET,

OUR EXERCISE HABITS

OUR ENVIRONMENT.

THERE IS NO FAT GENE.

Sorry, peeps. Especially if you'd chosen to hang your hat on that one as the reason why you're the way you are.

It's what you do to your genes that will make you fat –

OR NOT.

Your children's genetic blueprint will be set at conception according to the way your genes are expressing themselves at that time (mums and dads!). So, while there is no fat gene,

YOUR GENETIC EXPRESSION WILL BE HANDED OVER

to the next generation.

If you've been looking after those genes of yours, then your kids and their kids will **OWE YOU BIG TIME!**

COOL, HUH?

EXERCISING WHILE PREGNANT.

PART ONE

I love to see women training for the 'main event', as fitness is a valuable commodity during childbirth. It's always important to follow the advice of your doctor, though, so speak to them about it.

When it comes to exercise, the first trimester in pregnancy is all about

NOT OVERHEATING.

If you're a regular exerciser, you should be fine to continue, just at a less intense rate. **BUT** non-exercisers really need to take a steady and slow pace.

EXERCISING WHILE PREGNANT.

PART TWO

During pregnancy, you need to stop using your heart rate as a measure of exertion – your resting heart rate increases when you're expecting.

THERE'S ONLY ONE THING WORSE
THAN A HOLIDAY HANGOVER

– a holiday hangover when there's an extra three or four kilos of you pining to be back on the poolside sun lounge or carving your way down one of Niseko's wide runs.

Keep training on holidays, but don't fall into the trap of expecting killer work-outs and obliterated PBs (personal bests). You're in

MAINTENANCE MODE

while you're away – the aim is solely to come back the same weight you were in the taxi to the airport.

I'm always hearing

'BUT I TRAVEL FOR WORK!'

as the reason why someone can't get their act together with health and fitness.

Honestly, I have to say that I actually find it **EASIER** when I travel! I can order nutritious meals that someone else cooks, and I'm not at home doing everything that 'needs doing', giving me more time to train.

IT'S ACTUALLY THE BEST TIME TO GET INTO IT!

If you're travelling for work and staying in a big hotel, always order breakfast delivered to your room. The **ALL-YOU-CAN-EAT BUFFETS ARE RIDICULOUS** and way too tempting, especially if you're going to be sitting on your butt all day in meetings.

Choose fruit and yoghurt or a healthy cereal with skim milk, or a boiled egg with a multigrain toast – no butter.

YOU DON'T NEED TO EAT LIKE A SIX-FOOT LUMBERJACK.

ORDER AN EXTRA APPLE or two with breakfast. That way, when those dumb cakes, muffins and pastries come out at morning tea, you have an alternative. Really, who needs to be eating that

GARBAGE

when you're trying to work, think and stay awake?

AVOID EVENING DRINKING SESSIONS

when travelling for work. Be a grown-up. **BE WISE.** Leave the big nights out for the losers who'll be late and hung-over at the first meeting, unable to string a sentence together.

WAY TO GO TO GET THAT PROMOTION!

NOTHING,

BUT NOTHING,

PACKS ON THE KILOS LIKE ALCOHOL

and all the dumb food choices that go with it. Think about it – when was the last time you were **QUEUING FOR A KEBAB** at 2 a.m. sober?

Set yourself some rules before you go out, and intersperse alcoholic drinks with non-alcoholic ones.

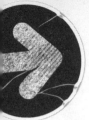

IT ALL STARTS WITH YOU.

The road to better health, better fitness, weight loss and better relationships is like any road to **TRUE** and lasting change. There are no shortcuts. You can't take the sneaky backstreet way. Trust me, that leads to disappointment, despair and frustration.

The **QUICK FIX** approach never works. If you're not prepared to pay the price, making what I call 'deposits in the bank' – smart choices about your food and exercise every day, consistently – you'll never achieve lasting change. Worse yet, you'll end up feeling empty, frustrated and powerless. Understandably, this can lead to the feeling that it's not you, it's them – **'IT'S NOT MY FAULT!'** The victim mentality can start to weave its sneaky way into your mindset, **WHICH HELPS NO ONE.**

Nope, you just can't obtain true, lasting, deep change unless you're prepared to travel the road daily, do the time and look within.

Rather than trying to bandaid the problem, look for its root. **THIS REQUIRES GUTS.** It requires you to live by some important yet powerful principles. Honesty. Commitment. Integrity. Respect. And it's a struggle. I struggle every day to live by these principles (and a few others I set for myself). At times I don't get it right, yet I truly believe that these are streetlights along the road to true change and bring with them a very rewarding and empowering life. My nan used to always say to me, 'Don't lower yourself to being someone who's consistently asking *What can I have?* If you want to create change, ask instead, *Who can I be?*' You can create change by *being* more –

MORE HONEST, MORE RESPONSIBLE, MORE YOUR WORD.

PENGUIN BOOKS

Published by the Penguin Group
Penguin Group (Australia)
250 Camberwell Road, Camberwell, Victoria 3124, Australia
(a division of Pearson Australia Group Pty Ltd)
Penguin Group (USA) Inc.
375 Hudson Street, New York, New York 10014, USA
Penguin Group (Canada)
90 Eglinton Avenue East, Suite 700, Toronto, Canada ON M4P 2Y3
(a division of Pearson Penguin Canada Inc.)
Penguin Books Ltd
80 Strand, London WC2R 0RL, England
Penguin Ireland
25 St Stephen's Green, Dublin 2, Ireland
(a division of Penguin Books Ltd)
Penguin Books India Pvt Ltd
11 Community Centre, Panchsheel Park, New Delhi – 110 017, India
Penguin Group (NZ)
67 Apollo Drive, Rosedale, North Shore 0632, New Zealand
(a division of Pearson New Zealand Ltd)
Penguin Books (South Africa) (Pty) Ltd
24 Sturdee Avenue, Rosebank, Johannesburg 2196, South Africa

Penguin Books Ltd, Registered Offices: 80 Strand, London WC2R 0RL, England

First published by Penguin Group (Australia), 2011

10 9 8 7 6 5 4 3 2 1

Text copyright © Michelle Bridges 2011

The moral right of the author has been asserted

Cover and text design by Adam Laszczuk © Penguin Group (Australia)
Cover photograph by Nick Wilson
Typeset in Chaparral Pro by Vanessa Battersby © Penguin Group (Australia)
Printed and bound in Australia by McPherson's Printing Group, Maryborough, Victoria

National Library of Australia Cataloguing-in-Publication data:

Bridges, Michelle.
Five minutes a day : Simple tips for weight-loss and wellbeing / Michelle Bridges.
9780143567059 (pbk.)
Health promotion. Fitness.

613.7

penguin.com.au

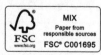